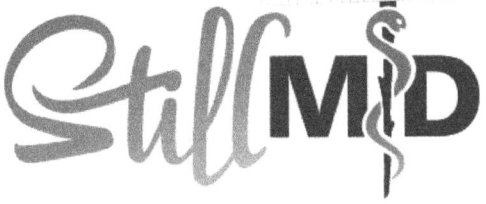

Two Physicians' Advice for International Medical Students & Graduates

Nina Lum, MD

Kimberly M. Brown, MD, MPH

Dr. Nina Lum's books and products are available at www.drninalum.com.

For more information, contact her directly at: ninalum@gmail.com

Dr. Kimberly Brown's books and products are available through online retailers and www.drkimberlybrownmd.com.

For more information, contact her directly at: info@drkimberlybrownmd.com

www.stillmd.com

ISBN 978-1-7330849-3-2

Still MD

DEDICATION

Dr. Lum

*To all the International Medical Graduates
(affectionately known as IMGs) I have met, inspired,
and led and for those I am yet to meet.*

Dr. Brown

*To those who crisscross the world in order to obtain the
knowledge needed to save lives.*

TABLE OF CONTENTS

GLOSSARY

AAMC: American Association of Medical Colleges

AMA: American Medical Association

CMS: Caribbean Medical Student/School

COMP: NBME Comprehensive Basic Science Exam

DO: Doctor of Osteopathic Medicine

ECFMG: Educational Commission for Foreign Medical Graduates

ERAS: Electronic Residency Application Service

FMG: Foreign Medical Graduate

FREIDA Online: Fellowship and Residency Electronic Interactive Database

IMG: International Medical Graduate

MCAT: Medical College Admission Test

MD: Medical Doctor

NBME: National Board of Medical Examiners

Non-US IMG: non-US citizen International Medical Graduate

NRMP: National Residency Match Program

US IMG: US citizen International Medical Graduate

US: United States

USA: United States of America

USMLE: United States Medical Licensure Examination

INTRODUCTION

I did not plan to go to a Caribbean medical school. Unlike Dr. Brown, I "stumbled upon" this alternative to practicing medicine in the United States after missing the only option available to me in my home country Cameroon in 2004.

To my dismay, according to the 2011 article in "US NEWS" magazine, Caribbean medical schools have been branded as the pathway for "weaker medical school applicants" over the years.[1] This concept was one that was oblivious to me when I chose this route.

According to the American Medical Association (AMA), IMGs make up 25% of the physician workforce in the US, a level of participation that has increased from 18 percent in 1970 and only 10

---

[1] https://www.usnews.com/education/blogs/medical-school-admissions-doctor/2011/08/01/pros-and-cons-of-applying-to-foreign-medical-schools

percent in 1963.[2] As an alumnus of the great blue seas now, I understand the hesitancy by many to accept physicians like myself as apt and "equals" to our 100 percent US-educated counterparts. By virtue of this knowledge, I, and the thousands who have gone before me, have worked hard to defy the negative stereotype associated with physicians who graduated from foreign medical schools.

I have dedicated the last four years since completing family medicine residency to consulting and coaching graduates of foreign medical schools on how to succeed in this current climate. As a person affectionately known in the medical community as an IMG, I work hard and continue to learn the expertise of primary care so that I can best serve my patients with the highest-quality standards available in the US healthcare market. My status as an IMG never comes up in the workplace itself; what matters today are my clinical acumen, board certification, work ethic, and bedside manner, among other things.

I wrote this book to help you with actionable steps you can take to create your success as an IMG. I have witnessed this same vigor I carry each time I've interviewed countless US and non-US IMGs for my blog series titled the "IMG Roadmap Series" on www.

2 American Medical Association, *Physician Characteristics and Distribution in the U.S.,* 2006 ed. (Chicago: AMA, 2006) Medline; and E.S. Salsberg and G.J. Forte, "Trends in the Physician Workforce, 1980–2000," *Health Affairs 21*, no. 5 (2002): 165–173. Medline, Google Scholar.

<u>theencouragingdoc.com</u>, a place where previous IMGs share success pearls on their nontraditional path to medicine. My conclusion today is that a great physician is made not only through the educational system they are reared in but the strength of their individual work ethic and devotion to high-value patient care in whatever plane of medicine that they choose.

Hopefully you, the foreign or international medical graduate that reads this book, will remember that *you* get to define your future and no one else can do that for you. The instruction in this book is meant to lead and guide you to do what other successful IMGs knew to do. Remember, "the end of a thing is better than the beginning thereof" – Ecclesiastes 8:7.

I am still an MD … ain't I?

Dr. Nina Lum

Nina and I met each other at a conference for women physicians in Atlanta, GA. I connected with her immediately. As we got to know each other, I realized we shared a similar journey into medicine, as we were both educated in Caribbean medical schools. I admired her pride and advocacy for other IMGs in being successful in medical school and residency.

To be very honest, for a long time, I was ashamed of the path that I took to become a physician. My whole life, everyone knew that I wanted to be a doctor, and I worked towards that goal diligently. To not go to a US medical school felt as though I was somehow less than someone that was educated stateside. After finishing my pre-clinicals in Dominica and coming back stateside, I'd compare myself to US medical students that I interacted with. I was always worried that they knew and had more than I did. During my first few months of residency, I struggled to ask questions because I was worried that everyone else knew the answer since I was the only foreign graduate in my program.

It took a while for me to be proud of the journey that I took to medicine. This route is definitely the road less traveled, and in some ways, it may be rougher. Looking back, however, taking the scenic route made me a better physician. I've treated people with almost no resources as well as every resource. Going to an offshore school built up my determination and resilience.

Dr. Nina and I wanted to share our experiences in order for you to know the road may be difficult, but it is not impossible. You may have a similar journey to me, as a US student considering going to, or actually being in, a Caribbean school. Or you may come from another country and decide to educate yourself in the Caribbean or another international medical school. The hope Dr. Nina and I have is that you can find similarities in our experiences and find inspiration in our stories.

After all, you're still an MD … right?

Dr. Kimberly Brown

CHAPTER 1

The Hustle Before the MD

Dr. Kim

I always wanted to become a doctor. My mother always says that I inherited her passion to become a physician, a passion she never got to fulfill. My mom wanted to be a doctor and be a mom and have five children. My dreams weren't so aggressive, but I definitely wanted to be a physician.

Throughout my years of growing up, my wanting to become a doctor flourished. At some point, I wanted to be a heart surgeon, at others I wanted to be an

OB-GYN or a forensic pathologist, but the point remains that I wanted to become a doctor. I attended college at Fisk University in Nashville, Tennessee, which is directly across the street from Meharry Medical College, a historically Black medical school. I was a pre-med/biology major, and Fisk had a joint program with Meharry that guaranteed acceptance into Meharry if I scored well on my MCAT and kept up a certain GPA. While I was at Fisk, it would pay for my tuition and fees. As someone who had difficulty paying for her first year at Fisk, the joint program was a huge opportunity.

I gained acceptance in the joint program and spent my sophomore and junior year at Fisk, working hard to keep my grades up. However, what I wasn't prepared for was the MCAT. The summer when I was supposed to be taking my MCAT I was studying but not doing well on my practice tests. When I took the actual MCAT, not surprisingly I didn't score well. I was dropped from the program.

Discouraged because all of my other pre-med friends had gotten into medical school, I ended up working and trying to decide my next moves. I took an MCAT prep class, worked, and had a social life, but still my scores weren't going anywhere. I began to become very discouraged. Around that time, I applied for the University of Florida's Master of Public Health program. I had learned about public health early on in undergrad, and I loved the idea of learning how systems affected individual health and how I could use that information to become a better physician. So I took my Graduate Reasoning Exam (GRE) It was much easier than the MCAT! Later, I was accepted to the University of Florida to study public health.

My first year in Florida went well. I did very well in my classes and was able to spend a month in Quito, Ecuador. I focused on learning medical Spanish, understanding the public health system in Ecuador and gaining clinical experience to put on my medical school application. In Ecuador, I discovered emergency medicine, and I changed my mind from becoming an OB-GYN, to becoming an emergency physician.

However, I was still stuck with one main problem. I had to get into medical school. By the beginning of the second year of my program, I had taken the MCAT a total of three times, each with horrible results. I didn't know to raise my score. I decided to apply to medical school again, more broadly than I had before. I picked up extra hours at my part-time job to cover the cost.

Again, almost like clockwork, the rejections started to roll in. I started sinking into a depression. I was getting multiple rejections from multiple schools. I was really frustrated and sad. All I'd ever wanted to be in life was to be a physician, but every time I applied to medical school or took the MCAT, I met failure and rejection.

One day, I was sitting on a friend's couch. I ended up telling him how sad and frustrated I was about getting rejected. He asked me if I had applied to Caribbean schools. I'd considered applying to a Caribbean school but I had so many hesitations. I worried about moving out of the country, possibly learning a new language—but, more importantly, I was afraid of the stigma that seemed to be attached to US residents going to school in the Caribbean. I'd heard other students talk negatively about students going to Caribbean schools and how they were not smart enough to get into medical school stateside.

My friend leveled with me. He had multiple friends that were practicing physicians that had gone to a Caribbean medical school, gotten into residency, and were successful. He told me if I was really passionate about being a physician, even by not getting in through the traditional American-school route, then I should just go ahead and apply to a Caribbean school. I thought about it long and hard.

By this time, I had several college friends who were at Ross University in Dominica. They were on the island, posting pictures talking about parties after exams, posting their successes moving through the semesters. I started to take a serious look at the websites of Ross, St. George's, and the American University of the Caribbean. I researched the islands they were on. Slowly but surely, I started to warm up to the idea of attending a Caribbean medical school. I reached out to one of my friends and had a Skype conversation with her about Ross, about medical school and life on the island. She addressed my biggest fears when she confirmed that everything was in English, that most students after graduating got into US schools, that third-year rotations were in the US. I realize at that point I had absolutely nothing to lose and everything to gain, so I went ahead and I submitted an application to Ross.

In January 2010, I was invited to interview! This was my first medical school invitation ever. After an in-person interview in Orlando, Florida—almost immediately after I interviewed—I took a long drive to Washington, DC to start an internship to finish my public health degree. A few weeks later, I got some amazing news. I was accepted into the January 2011 starting semester at Ross University School of Medicine! I finished my internship in DC, drove back to Florida, presented my final research, and graduated in May 2010.

The countdown began ... I had only six months until I would have to be in Dominica to start a new journey in a brand new country.

DR. NINA

I am among the minority group of US-based physicians who did not take the MCAT. Neither am I the traditional IMG. You may be wondering how that is the case because, for the most part, being a graduate of a foreign medical school is nontraditional enough. I actually learned about this seemingly terrifying examination while already a medical student rotating at a hospital on Chicago's South Side during my third year of medical school.

Yes, as a Caribbean medical student, the third- and fourth-year curricula of medical school are typically completed at a US hospital(s). Though my background may be atypical of the average American, my current results and achievements are on par with my US counterparts today.

Born and raised in the armpit of Africa's western coastline, my knowledge of America was one founded on media and magazines. It is no surprise then when I tell you that the educational system and structure were not familiar to me either. With my mother being a pediatrician, medicine was the way of life. My brother and I spent our summers working odd jobs in her private practice. This woman took no breaks from work and no traditional vacations except for medical leave. She is of the prior generation of medical professionals where no duty hours existed. (Duty hours are recent regulations placed on the graduate medical education system in the US to limit the hours spent by physicians in training.)

Back to Mom. Medicine is still a part of our family. My father helped her build a structure you might best imagine as a "she shed" on the property of our home for neighborhood consults. This was in addition to the other two clinical jobs Mom kept up throughout my childhood. I was immensely inspired by her work. The impact she had on the community was unmatched, especially in a country with a shortage of pediatricians and physicians in general. This inspiration led me to transfer my credits from my undergraduate coursework in microbiology at the only English university in Cameroon, at the time, to a pre-medical program in Curacao, from which I eventually matriculated into medical school at the same institution.

But your path will be different from mine because that is the characteristic of the journey to every professional career. One article in the "Health Affair" journal showed that there has been a steady increase in the number of ECFMG applicants attending medical schools in the Caribbean. In 1992, 321 US IMG applicants attended a medical school located somewhere in the Caribbean, representing 41.7 percent of the US IMG applicant pool in that year; in 2006, 1,966 applicants—nearly 71 percent of all US citizen applicants—did so.[3] That being said, no two physicians share the same stories because subtle variances always exist. Other factors, such as financial constraints, academic background, personal performance, country of citizenship, and even mindsets differ between applicants.

Knowing this, I am certain you may either be in the process of going to a foreign school or may have recently matriculated into one, or maybe you already graduated from one but are looking to revise or to advise someone else. If you are reading this book, you are more likely to be debating this "scenic" option. So here are a few directional points to consider.

• Research your personal options

… for transitioning back to the US before you go to a foreign medical school. It is important to understand the odds of success with this journey. Be willing to take risks and be cognizant of the consequences. It is no surprise that there are more unmatched graduates from foreign medical schools than there are from US schools.

3 https://www.healthaffairs.org/doi/full/10.1377/
hlthaff.28.1.226#R1 TRENDS U.S. Citizens Who Obtain Their
Medical Degrees Abroad: An Overview, 1992–2006. John R. Boulet,
Richard A. Cooper, Stephen S. Seeling, John J. Norcini, Danette W.
McKinley.

- **Define your reason for taking this route**

You do not know what you do not know. Start your research early enough. Create a purpose statement, because medical school is going to be one of the most trying experiences of your life. You better be clear about it so you do not give up when the road gets tough.

- **Research your route**

It is imperative to gather as much information before you make the next step because this single decision can make or break your chances of practicing medicine as a whole. In this section, I have some questions for you to answer. This is like you giving yourself much-needed introspection before you begin this journey. I recommend you write down your responses as you work through this section. I hope your dream of practicing medicine quickly shifts from a dream to a goal by the end of this chapter.

- **Define and reconsider your "why"**

The four years required to complete medical school will be challenging, and you may discover the unique factors that delineate a successful graduate from a foreign medical school from their unsuccessful counterparts. But you do not want to learn this through personal experience! So you need a strong reason why you want this, then an action plan as to how you will make it through. A key thing to consider throughout this journey is your eventual chances of matching into a US residency. This should be quickly followed by your chances for matching into a competitive specialty and then what opportunities may become readily available to you when you complete training to become an attending physician. But one step at a time.

- **Identify your purpose for pursuing this path**

Questions to ask yourself:

- Is this a financial decision?
- Is this a viable option for you?
- Do you know what you might possibly be interested in specializing in?
- Do you have a mentor or someone who has done what you are wanting to do?

- **Build your "gusto"**

It was my observation that several of my medical schoolmates dropped out along the way. I believe when there weren't any unforeseen circumstances, such as health issues or death, this was because they had no "gusto" to begin with. When medicine is the only thing you see yourself doing, you should find it even harder to give up. Perseverance is the secret recipe to the taking the nontraditional route to medicine. Your perseverance through the process will build you up for what lies ahead. You have to keep being consistent in showing up to class, in creating extra time to study by eliminating unnecessary tasks and you will find yourself on the other side of your dream.

• Consider your alternative(s)

"Why am I not going to a US medical school?" If you do not have a clear response to this question, pause and continue this exercise with me.

You should be able to stratify this based on certain factors. Included but not limited to:

- Financial – "I cannot afford it."

- Educational Performance – "I did not do competitively well on the MCAT" or "I do not qualify for the schools in my area" or " I was rejected from the medical schools I applied to."

- Mental – " I just can't do it." This is usually based on self-imposed limitations that have nothing to do with your future academic potential but are founded on traumas, fears, and limitations from our upbringing or prior experiences in school and within our communities.

When US undergraduate students contact me with questions about whether they should go to foreign schools, my instinctive response is a resounding "NO"—unless they have clearly evaluated all these reasons listed above.

• Analyze the end from the beginning

If you have the luxury of knowing exactly what you want to specialize in, then this is always best. But for many of us, we allowed medical school to expose us to our options. Considering that the most competitive specialties tend to have the fewest number of IMGs to train, if you are hoping to be a neurosurgeon, an orthopedist, or a dermatologist, you may find it easier studying in the USA as research and mentorship really make a marked difference in acceptance into these fields. Being an offshore school with few alumni following this path may prove to be a hindrance. A December 2018 article published on the AMA website showed that pathology, internal medicine, neurology, and family medicine were among the most friendly IMG specialties. They quoted percentages of IMGs that matched into these specialties for that year to be: pathology 46.2%, internal medicine 43.2%, neurology 35%, and family medicine 30.3 %.[4] Knowing that past performance is predictive of future outcomes, you may want to analyze "your possible end" from the beginning using these odds. If you are okay with the statistics, then keep going.

4 https://www.ama-assn.org/residents-students/specialty-profiles/4-medical-specialties-among-friendliest-img-pgy-1-matches by Brendan Murphy, AMA News Writer.

CHAPTER 2

Before You Take Off ...

DR. KIM

After I finished my master's program, I moved back home to Milwaukee, Wisconsin, experiencing my home city for the first time as an adult. I found a job working for a local social-services agency, doing a mix of public health and social work. And I loved it! My job was to help Wisconsin Medicaid recipients understand how to use their benefits, ensure children had the appropriate screenings, and connect them with any other needs they may have had. The hours were long, but I left work daily knowing that I helped someone. Although I loved the job, I didn't make very much, and balancing paying bills and preparing to live outside of the US was hard. I had to pay for visas, an admission deposit, summer clothes (I was going to live in a tropical climate year-round), plane tickets to Dominica, school supplies, and medical diagnosis equipment, then ship it to a different country. Things got expensive quickly. On top of that, I was keeping a huge secret from everyone at my job. No one knew I was going to medical school! I couldn't tell anyone that I had just started the job but now I would be leaving at the first of the year.

Outside of work and preparing to leave, I had a lot of stressors in my personal life. Tensions began to grow within my family, and I started to feel unsupported. I had someone extremely close to me as I grew up pass away after a long illness. Also, I dealt with my own personal health issues. Earlier in the year, my father passed away and I started to deal with the emotions regarding his loss. It just seemed like the world crashed around me right before I was taking the huge leap to start a new journey.

Out of all of the research that I did before I was accepted to Ross, very few people talked about the emotional journey it can be. Although I had lived out of the country for one month, moving to live in another country for two years is very different. Family and friends are far away, you are immersed in a new place, culture, and maybe even a language that you may or may not be comfortable with. And that's hard. On top of that, you are about to be in a rigorous educational program that will consume a lot of time and energy.

With that all being said, here's what I think you should know, which maybe no one else will tell you, before you go.

- It's okay to be scared. This is a monumental feat that most people don't understand the bravery that it takes to do. Medical school is challenging, but doing it in another country can be even more challenging. Allow yourself to feel the jitters—you've got this!

- Build a support system and lean on it. Although you may be in a different time zone than your family and friends, it's still important to keep in touch with them. Social media is a great way to connect, but sometimes it can be too much of a distraction. Try to plan to make time for your family and friends by scheduling calls on a regular basis, like after exams. It's easy to get wrapped up with the day-to-day hectic schedule of school, but having a regular time to connect with loved ones is important.

- Get the negative stereotypes and thoughts around Caribbean medical school out of your head. You're going to get an amazing education if you work hard and pursue your dream. Every school has the tools you need to help you to succeed, like tutoring for example.

- Get to know as much as possible about the area

outside of the school. I didn't know that the island of Dominica existed before I considered applying to Ross. Before I went, I took some time to do some research on the island, to understand the native language, culture, and possible things to do while I was there. It definitely eased my transition: I knew exactly what to expect once I landed.

Dr. Nina

For a girl who failed the medical school entrance exam in Cameroon in 2004, I showed up without hesitation at the only airport in my hometown. Cheesy as it sounds, I wasn't going to miss a flight to my dreams.

But nothing could prepare me for where I am today. The road ahead could have seemed daunting to other eighteen-year-old girls, but to me on this beautiful day in June, this was a pivotal journey. I was about to soar into my destiny, oblivious to the significance of the ECFMG, USMLE exams or the prejudice faced by other graduates of foreign medical schools in America.

But then again, I was not flying to America. I was headed to the island of Curacao to complete a pre-medical curriculum, with no idea that I would end up practicing here in the States.

As an early career hospital medicine physician today, when I reflect back there wasn't a point in time where I thought about the societal honor bestowed on my future by virtue of being a physician. Neither did I ever, even for a second, consider the potential financial compensation that could come from a future practicing general medicine. I just wanted to become a doctor. As an undergraduate student studying in the department of "Life Sciences" at the only English university in Cameroon, I majored in microbiology. I dreamed about medicine in its traditional sense—

Primary care. And here I was flying closer to that dream. Thinking about that now, I was completely ignorant as to the responsibility which I now hold with this title.

Ignorance is bliss, they say. I walked through the Douala International Airport, accompanied by my uncle who worked there. Vested in his light-green hazmat suit and helmet, he was my mouthpiece as we went through check-in, security, immigration, and then some more security.

The engines of the airplanes roared like something out of a sci-fi nightmare. I clenched my fist firmly on the seat handles, almost touching my uncaring neighbor, who was unbothered by the process of taking off. But this moment metaphorically painted the emotions I would feel before every test, every new rotation, every residency interview. A nervous trepidation at the thought of failure. My first takeoff was terrifying enough, but what was most terrifying to me was that I had a valid Cameroonian passport without a visa stamp in it. The thought of deportation once I arrived at the island filled my head. For most Americans, visas are not an issue due to global entry and worldwide reciprocities that facilitate this process. But for West Africans, a visa can make or break your goal if travel is a means to its end.

Before a plane takes off, it has to rise up against a gravitational pull. The wings of the plane need to generate enough difference in turbulence between the top and the bottom blades to keep the currents that allow this massive bird to cut through skies with divine precision.

In many ways, when a student chooses to pursue a competitive yet challenging career path in medicine, they experience a pullback—typically in the form of all the reasons why they cannot do that what they so desire. Are you going to take charge and create the opposing force to keep your dream afloat?

Before you take off, consider these:

- Verify entry requirements to the island, especially non-US citizens, as these vary with narrower options for non-US citizens. Most islands allow US citizens entry without a visa, but each island may require a "residence permit" for the duration of your extended time on the island. Request additional information from island authorities prior to leaving the US.

- Investigate the school's accreditation status. (This may not apply to the four foundational schools that have been around for decades. Each country in the Caribbean and the world may have different accrediting agencies.). Accreditation is the process of ensuring educational quality. For schools located in the Caribbean, accreditation is a key component in your future education. It will determine issues such as your eligibility to sit the USMLE and/or subsequent eligibility to become certified by the Educational Commission for Foreign Medical Graduates.

- The LCME (Liaison Committee on Medical Education: jointly sponsored by the AAMC & AMA) is the US accrediting body for programs leading to the MD degree in the United States.[5] For osteopathic schools, the equivalent is the Commission of Osteopathic College Accreditation (for DO schools).[6] When looking for Caribbean schools, search for schools that carry the accreditations approved by the LCME.

- FAIMER[7] (Foundation for Advancement of International Medical Education and Research) is NOT an accrediting agency, but it does provide a Directory of Organizations that Recognize/ Accredit Medical Schools (DORA). Use the DORA site to look up the organization that accredits schools for the island of your choice and then ask your school whether they have the appropriate accreditation stated. This should only be a "yes" or "no" response. Remember that a government charter and/or being listed in a

5 https://www.aamc.org/members/osr/committees/48814/reports_lcme.html

6 http://www.osteopathic.org/inside-aoa/accreditation/COM-accreditation/Pages/default.aspx

7 https://www.faimer.org/resources/dora/index.html

medical school directory (e.g., World Directory of Medical Schools, FAIMER, IMED, WHO) is NOT the same as being accredited. Again, refer to accreditation above and note the ONLY agencies that can offer such services.

- Avoid schools that do not have a track record of success. If the school does not have alumni doing what you want to do, it is probably not the safest choice for you. Consider that there are several other credible schools located on the islands that can offer you better education and have graduated residents from training programs in America for decades. You should expect the past successful performance of the school to be on par with what you can potentially get. It is no surprise that several foreign medical schools have emerged from businessmen seeking long-term monetary gain. Beware of such schools preying on your dreams.

- Verify connections between your school and US clinical rotation sites and also whether your school will provide support for your US visa application when the time comes for clinical rotations.

- For students from non-US undergraduate schools who have not completed a degree program, ensure your coursework credits are assessed by a reputable US-based evaluator. Have your credits evaluated and made acceptable to US standards prior to embarking on this journey to the Caribbean as it is required you attend medical school after completion of an undergraduate degree in the US. This differs from other European and African curricula, where medical school entrance occurs right after high school.

- Other credibility & reputation. Research, research, research. Talk to alumni, current students, etc. Look up the school's social media platform to see what the students are really saying. Call the island authorities. Do whatever you need to do to get information on the consistency of faculty members, availability of laboratory resources, medical libraries, necessary amenities, etc. Question opportunities for research and also the availability of reputable spots for clinical rotations during third and fourth years. With the recent wave of natural disasters, while weather shouldn't be a limiting factor, sporadic and destructively bad weather can happen anywhere, so you should certainly consider it.

- Investigate options for financial aid that are available to US citizens and non-US citizens (the possibility of a US citizen cosigner may exist in some cases).

CHAPTER 3

Welcome to the Jungle

Dr. Kim

Getting to Dominica was nothing short of a disaster. I'd bought my ticket months prior from a discount travel website (that is no longer in service). My flight took me from Milwaukee to New Jersey, where I had a long layover, then on to Trinidad and Trinidad to Dominica. I was extremely nervous, but I was on my way. I went to New Jersey and met up with some family, who showed me around. They dropped me off at the airport later in the day. When I landed in Trinidad, I found a busy and bustling airport. I had a voicemail on my phone telling me to call the now-out-of-service discount airline-finding company. I was afraid to call back because I was too broke to make international calls. Instead, I kept looking over and over for my airline. I couldn't find it anywhere. I asked a representative from another airline where the stall was; she couldn't tell me. I asked someone else. They said that the airline was out of business. Out of business? After a few more minutes of insanity, I gave up looking for the airline and bit the bullet to make the international call.

After quite some time, I learned that, at the last minute, my flight from Trinidad to Dominica had been canceled because the airline went out of business. The booking company had called minutes before my flight was to take off to let me know that my flight had been canceled. There was no way to rebook me. I was stranded.

I was a broke, *almost* Caribbean medical student with NO money, stranded in another country.

I had no one to call. I had family problems at home, so I couldn't call my immediate family. I felt very alone. I put a status on Facebook about my plight of being stranded in Trinidad. A few minutes later, my aunt commented on my status. After messaging her and calling her, she bought me a flight to Dominica. I had enough money for maybe a hotel room, but definitely not a flight and a place to stay. I found an inexpensive bed and breakfast to stay in, made a call, and they picked me up from the airport.

In the morning, I was on my way from Trinidad to Dominica on a tiny little LIAT (the Caribbean airline) plane.

Dr. Nina gives some great advice below about planning ahead for your time on the island regarding housing and academics. Your school will likely send more information about obtaining a student visa. I'd add the following tips:

- Be prepared for an emergency. Emergencies in the sense of finances and environment. As you prepare to head to the island, try to save a small amount of money in case you need to exit the island due to bad weather or personal emergency. Consider having flashlights, candles, portable chargers for cell phones and electronic devices with you as you pack to go.

- Consider arriving early on the island to get acclimated. There is a lot to explore on the island before you are busied with the rigors of classes. There are usually some other students hanging around, and it's a great way to meet new people.

- Try to send as little ahead as possible. So many students worry about shipping food, clothing, and electronics ahead of them. I sent all of the above, including a printer. In hindsight, I needed a quarter of what I sent ahead. In the end, I wasted a lot of money, and I had too many things to worry about shipping back to the US when

I was finished with my basic sciences. Consider packing to take with you or shipping ahead:

- **External hard drive**

- **Office supplies (printer paper, colored pens, highlighters, sticky notes, etc.)**

- **Your favorite non-perishable/shelf-stable foods/snacks that you can't live without**

Everything else can wait. Give yourself the time on the island to find out what you absolutely are missing and consider shipping it to yourself the next semester.

Dr. Nina

Jan was a rare breed. A Belgian-Congolese that lived on the island of Curacao for several years and worked at my future school. It was comforting to hear someone familiar welcoming me on arrival at the Curacao International Airport: "Bienvenue, Nina!" What were the odds that I would meet a francophone West African over five thousand miles away, I thought to myself! I was elated to hear a familiar language.

The views of Curacao from the airport were the most breathtaking. We rode back to the Plaza Hotel, where I was going to stay until I could find more affordable housing on the island. This was only the beginning of a beautiful struggle.

Here is what I suggest you need to know about arriving on the island:

- Plan ahead for housing: seek out students who will be starting with you and buddy up as roommates. You want to be fully settled before school starts, so show up earlier if you can to sort out these details. Island housing is a lot more affordable when compared to housing in America, so this can be a place to save money if finances are limited.

- Along with planning for housing, also seek out the recommended textbooks for the first semester so you can purchase at a discount from other students or from Amazon prior to embarking on your journey to the island. You want to be prepared prior to your first day of school as opposed to seeking out PDF resources once classes begin.

- If you delay in preparing, let me tell you this: you are always going to be behind. So, seek out resources from your seniors, ask about the structure of classes, investigate the recommended texts or other resources. Prepare to start early. This seems like I'm being repetitive, I know. But many students arrive on the island unprepared for medical school. I say you begin your work on USMLE Step 1 on the *first day* of school. The biggest mistake you can make is waiting until the end of the basic science semesters before you begin to think about a plan for USMLE Step 1. The best way to address this is to remember that everything you learn during those first two years will determine your competitiveness for residency training in the States in the near future. So, do not screw yourself over before you even begin!

- As always, your safety and security come first. The legal atmosphere on the island may permit actions that would be considered as criminal in America to go unnoticed. It is up to you to make wise choices. We have all unfortunately heard horror stories of students who got entangled with drugs and alcohol. Others may have found themselves in the wrong place at the wrong time, and a few have even died while pursuing an offshore opportunity at a career in medicine. Please be careful with the company you choose to keep as you will be the sum total of all the people you surround yourself with.

- Find a routine that works: incorporate up to seven-eight hours of sleep, take care of yourself, incorporate exercise, and stay as healthy as possible. Adequate sleep hygiene seems to be one place where students struggle the most. Poor sleep can affect your cognitive function in class the following day. I recommend a routine that brings you to a library or quiet study spot after dinner, then setting a specific bedtime and adhering to it. I also found that I retained information a lot more when I studied early in the morning.

CHAPTER 4

Deep-sea Diving into the First Two Years

Dr. Kim

Dominica is a very interesting place. Black sand beaches, lush palm trees, winding roads. When they land, most people say it reminds them of Jurassic Park! All you can see is a very thick dense forest and you wonder if you're going to have to forage your way back to the campus. But all of a sudden, a clearing appears and you can see a landing strip and a very small airport waiting for you right alongside the ocean.

I miss a lot of things about Dominica. I loved going to the Shacks (an outdoor cafeteria area run by locals) and getting freshly squeezed guava juice, bake (a fried bread stuffed with meats and cheeses), lobster dinners, and crepes stuffed with savory things like pesto, cheese, and chicken. Making friends with each of the locals. Ordering delivery from Bob's Chinese. Splurging on Tomato's (an Americanesque restaurant) when I really needed something that tasted like home. Getting my nails done at Lindi's Nail Shop after exams. She was the only person on the island that had my favorite nail polish brand; it reminded me of being back in the States. For most of my first semester, we didn't have an actual grocery store near campus. Saturday mornings were trips to the Save-a-Lot in Roseau, an hour away from campus and a very winding, motion-sickness-inducing journey.

Despite all of the wonderful things that I found on the island, academically, I struggled my first semester. I had the same study habits in my first few weeks of medical school that I'd had my whole life. I studied at home, in my room, with the TV on and Facebook open. Needless to say, my first two exams weren't the best. I had always done well at everything in school, except for the MCAT. I figured if someone would look past that flaw, when I got to medical school it would be a breeze.

Well, it wasn't. When I got my scores back from my first exam, I was shocked. I'd never failed a test. I thought it was a fluke: failing was not something I was used to. The day I received my scores from the second exam, I completely freaked out. I cried to my study partner. All of these thoughts rushed into my head: "Maybe I'm not cut out to be a doctor. This isn't for me. I can't fail my very first semester of medical school, after everyone I've ever known knows that I want to be a doctor. I can't face the humiliation. What if I was wrong about myself?"

So I got desperate. Ross had a department called Academic Success (though I think they have since changed its name). Academic Success was a department that did … well, as the name suggests, ensure your academic success. Tutoring sessions, studying plans, small group sessions for review … You name it, they helped to make sure you had all of the tools, tips, and strategies to do well. A few of the faculty members made a presentation during orientation week and I half-listened. I'd never needed a tutor; obviously that was for dumb kids, I'd thought to myself.

I walked down to their offices and, holding back my tears, I asked to speak to a faculty member. I sat down with a counselor the next day and cried my eyes out. I told her that I was scared: I had failed my first two exams and I didn't know what I was doing wrong. After calming me down, she helped me come up with a plan to help me get on the right track, which included tutoring sessions, questions, a schedule, and skills to learn how to study. I literally did everything she said, starting the day I left her office. I worked hard, and the next exam, guess what? I did exceedingly well. I never failed another exam again.

After putting my academic struggles behind me, I tried my best to settle into island life. I had a lot of family drama at home, and I carried my family problems into my social life in Dominica. I had a hard time making friends, probably because I was struggling with things personally. I didn't know how to separate the two so I took things out on other people. Despite that, I do have really fun memories of the island, including traveling to my father's home country of Barbados, hanging out at the Shacks, our food-court area, long Skype conversations with family and friends back in the States, enjoying my three-times-a-week maid service, and enjoying laundry service as well.

When I could afford it, I would meet up with some friends at a hotel and resort on a hill and have brunch on Sunday mornings overlooking the rest of the island and campus. With nothing else modern on the island, Dominica had an incredible beauty to it that I enjoyed and now miss. When it rained, I'd open the windows in my apartment and enjoy the rain hitting the leaves on the banana trees. The downside of the rain in Dominica would be brown water coming from the shower, sinks, and toilet. Awful! Regardless, I'm very grateful that I was able to study medicine in another country and be able to focus on myself for sixteen months to pursue my goals.

I stayed in Dominica for my fifth semester, which was Ross University's bridge to our clinical years. Remaining in Dominica for fifth semester was the best thing I could have done for myself: not only was it less expensive than moving back stateside, but I was able to get so much more hands-on experience as an almost new third-year medical student than the other students did stateside. I was also able to build friendships with people that I hadn't gotten a chance to during the hubbub of the other semesters because we weren't in the same social circles or they had different routines or backgrounds. I was also able to focus on passing the COMP, otherwise known as the comprehensive exam. The COMP was used to help judge how much basic science knowledge we gained on the island; it was also a strong predictor of how well you'd do on USMLE Step 1. We were required to pass COMP in order to be approved to take Step 1. I didn't want to move back to the United States, get settled, and then study for another serious exam.

Lessons learned?

- **Never be afraid to say you don't know something or to ask for help.** When I decided to admit to myself that I had no clue what I was doing, that's when I was able to change my path. A lot of times, unexpected failure can lead to insanity, doing the same thing over and over but expecting a different result. I never believed that

I was "that person" that needed tutoring, extra help, or more study sessions. But soon I realized that this was a different game I was playing; one I had never played before. And if you have never played before, you need to know the rules of engagement to know how to win. It doesn't make you less smart to say, "I don't know" or "I need help." It makes you stronger and, eventually, will make you a better physician.

- **Lean on those who went before you.** At Ross, the Black Student Association had a mentorship program where second-semester students of color were paired with first-semester students. Your mentor took you under their wing and gave you the tools for success. This could be in the form of academic advice, companionship, a shoulder to cry on, and friendship. The times that I spent with my student mentors and later, mentees, helped to create an on-campus community that supported me while I was going through the rigors of the island. This isn't a competition or a sprint. It's a marathon, and you need a village.

- **Schedule. Schedule. Schedule.** What should you schedule? Everything! Class, gym time, sleeping, study hours, fun appointments, parties, organizational meetings ... Schedule it all. I liked to use Google Calendar, but if you're someone that prefers to manually write things down, get a written planner. In medical school, time is short and very precious. You need to know where your time is going so that you can plan appropriately. My basic science program was accelerated (sixteen months), so there was little time for extended breaks. Once an exam was taken and passed, the very next day we were starting a new organ system. Get on a schedule and stick to it ... If there is something you want to do, SCHEDULE it. And schedule your time off!

- **Get counseling/therapy to help with past/current issues to help you focus better on the goal ahead of you.** There is a lot of mental pressure that comes with medical school, especially when you leave your home country to attend. If things get overwhelming, do not stay silent. *Your* mental health is just as important as the health of your future patients. Reach out to someone at your school: they should be able to provide you with a counselor or a therapist to talk things through.

Dr. Nina

We took off sprinting. After completing my pre-medicine curriculum it was time to put on my big girl pants and chew the meat of the first semester of medical school. Between purchasing the recommended texts, moving into a new apartment, and the pressure of tuition starting to set in—not to mention the glorious smell of formaldehyde in the anatomy lab—I clearly was not mentally prepared. Before I knew it, I was partying to cope and dating to fill a void. Both were redeemed by the saving graces of my being an above-average test taker at this point in my life. These months were blurry; I do not recall much, but I do know every lesson I learned from this time and I will share them with you.

- Basic sciences are the most important years of your future as an IMG as the USMLE is still, in my opinion, the highest determining factor as to your chances of matching into a US residency or graduate medical-education program.

- Your goal of going to a Caribbean medical school is to match into a US residency program. According to the US program director's survey in 2018, 94% of program directors ranked the USMLE Step 1 score at a 4.1 mean importance rating for each factor in selecting applicants for interview (based on a scale of a low of 1 to a high of 5).[8] This means the people who make executive decisions about who gets admitted to residency training programs still deem your performance on the USMLE as a top-filtering criterion. This is exactly why specialties like plastic surgery and neurosurgery require higher scores than internal or family medicine.

• Skipping classes or using the Caribbean portion of your education as an extended vacation is not going to help you. You cannot rob yourself and expect to win. I recall some students being led astray by trying their hand at drugs or other illegal substances for recreation while on the island. If this is something you wouldn't do while enrolled in a US medical school, please do not do it while on the island either. You need to hold yourself to the same standard.

• Truth is, there is no easy way to success: not on an island, not skipping the MCAT to get the "easy way out." You will be held responsible for your actions, whether directly or indirectly. Believe that you only reap what you sow. So if you want to become a great physician, be a great student. Learn when presented the opportunity. Show up to every class, respect the pain of the process, repeat the class if that's what it takes. Taking a shortcut or asking for a curve to pass a

8 https://www.nrmp.org/wp-content/uploads/2018/07/NRMP-2018-Program-Director-Survey-for-WWW.pdf

class is still going to catch up with you later on when you can't seem to pass the pre-test needed to clear you to take the USMLE Step 1.

- I think it is important for me to share a little more on Dr. Kim's last point on seeking mental health help. Please seek therapy when you need it. At the beginning of my second year of medical school, I took advantage of a counseling service provided by my school. My interpersonal relationship with a senior medical student was unstable and it was beginning to affect my academic performance. The constant worry was a distraction to me. This mental health consultation saved me. It helped me manage stress, develop coping mechanisms and realign my perception of the situation. This allowed me to focus on what truly mattered at the time which was my education.

- In all, I want you to remember that there are no shortcuts to success—you have to do the work. The work may be academic, physical or mental but there is a sacrifice that has to made. It is often a sacrifice of time and effort but let me assure you that it will be worth it if you persevere.

CHAPTER 5

The Holy Grail: USMLE Step 1

DR. KIM

I left Dominica in August 2012 and headed back to Milwaukee to study for USMLE Step 1. It had been forever since I lived at home, and I missed EVERYTHING about the United States, especially my hometown favorite foods—and more importantly my car.

I did know that I needed to approach Step 1 with a lot of preparation and care. Trying to get into emergency medicine residency would be difficult as an IMG. I took about a week off before studying, and I booked my Step 1 for October 2012. After my week off, I put myself on a study schedule and I got back down to work. But being back stateside helped me to realize a couple of different things. Here's what I didn't anticipate.

- I didn't give myself enough time to relax and enjoy being back home. I needed more than just a week to settle back into living in the States ... especially after living abroad for almost twenty months!

- I didn't find a place to study outside of home. My room was small, crowded, and full of distractions from my family. I wish I had found a quiet coffee shop or library sooner to get work done.

- I didn't follow my own advice and schedule events that I wanted to attend around my study times. There were social events that I knew I wanted to go to now that I was stateside again. I often put my studying to the side in order to hang out.

After returning to the States (or your home country), it can be really easy to lose focus on what you have ahead: Step 1. Step 1 levels the playing field for medical students and future residency applicants, no matter what part of the globe they attended school. Here are several different ways that medical students can sabotage themselves when preparing for Step 1:

- **Underestimating the importance of the exam.**

No matter whether you went to Harvard, Yale or medical school X in the Caribbean, getting an amazing score on Step 1 puts you on par with everyone else across the world. The higher you score on Step 1, the greater the likelihood you'll have of successfully matching into a residency program.

- **Your environment.** You may be back stateside/home and suffer distractions from the convenience of living at home again.

- **Not sticking to your study plan or schedule.** It's very easy to think that you don't need to follow such a rigorous study schedule now that you're back stateside. You have more comforts of home, and your friends and family are not an ocean away. However, I found this time to be the most difficult because I was distracted by all of those things. It's much easier to stop doing practice questions because your friends want you to join them for Happy Hour. Remaining focused and dedicated to your schedule will take some work. Enlist other people's support by telling them how important this exam and your study schedule are to you.

- **Not setting a goal.** What's your dream score? Better yet, after you've done some research into your desired specialty, what is the average score of those matching into that specialty? Not sure? Then you should seek (of course), the highest score possible. No one gets a perfect "300." Keep your goal in mind while you are studying. I actually wrote it down and made a vision board around it. Whenever you get tired of studying or discouraged, remember your goal.

- **Not knowing when to take a break.** It's so easy to get obsessed with your dream score, sticking to a schedule, your dream specialty, or overcoming your mindset around going to school outside of the US. If you don't take scheduled breaks, it's easy to be overcome by stress and anxiety. TAKE A BREAK. Schedule time to hang out with friends, work out, attend religious services, practice yoga, take naps ... Whatever you need to do to maintain a healthy mental, social, spiritual, and physical balance while you are studying.

- **Not covering all the material.** If you have to take the NBME (National Board of Medical Examiners) Comprehensive Basic Science Exam, otherwise known as the COMP, it's easy to feel like you have everything covered in that study material more thoroughly than you actually have. As you are studying for Step 1, make sure you cover every bit of material.

- **Not going over the material that you're uncomfortable with or that you don't like.** I hate biochemistry! Sorry to all the biochem nerds out there. I hated it in college and in medical school. When it was time to cover it for Step 1, I ignored it and studied only what I liked and what made me comfortable. When I finally received my scores, my lowest section was—you guessed it—biochemistry. I could have easily scored higher if I took the time to review it more. Later, after I thought about the questions on my test, I realized they were straightforward! If I had taken a little time to go over the material, I'm certain I would have gotten those questions correct.

- **Not doing practice exams regularly.** You wouldn't go play in the World Cup without practicing, right? So why wouldn't you take a practice exam (or exams!) prior to taking Step 1? I took several practice exams to gauge where I was in my learning and how close I was to obtaining my dream score. I used the practice tests associated with the question banks I was using and also paid for NBME exams.

- **Using too many resources.** It's really easy in this day and age to get overwhelmed with different study programs that guarantee you certain scores. There are multiple question banks, review programs, podcasts, and audio programs. Way too much! My advice is to stick to a few different options and don't change. In order to be successful, you need to cover all of the material: use a question bank, and test yourself regularly to maintain your progress. When I studied for Step 1, I used Doctors in Training, UWorld Question Bank, Pathoma, as well as listening to Dr. Goljan audio in my spare time.

Dr. Nina

It was dusty, rowdy, and loud in Caracas, Venezuela. Everyone spoke so fast! The little Spanish I learned from Curacao over the previous twenty-four months of basic sciences was useless at this point. I could not communicate with anyone, but all I needed to do was present myself at the US embassy to obtain a visa to go to the US so I could participate in a Kaplan review course and sit for the USMLE Step 1 examination.

The hills of Caracas were a vision of the road ahead, torturous and unrevealing. Fast forward a few months later and here I am, facing the biggest test of my life as I sit for Step 1 in Cleveland, Ohio. After barely passing Step 1, I still did not understand that this was going to become a hindrance in the future. But the even bigger hindrance I would encounter was the fact that I required visa sponsorship to be accepted into any training programs. A double whammy! But I made it after all that, so here are a few pointers for you:

- Begin with the end in mind. Understand that the USMLE "is a three-step examination for medical licensure in the US The USMLE assesses a physician's ability to apply knowledge, concepts, and principles, and to demonstrate fundamental patient-centered skills, that are important in health and disease and that constitute the basis of safe and effective patient care."[9]

9 https://www.usmle.org/

- One study by Johnson et al. found that performance on exams throughout the first- and second-year curricula were highly correlated with scores on the Step 1 exams. Further, correlations were particularly high for those exams that had more components of physiology and/or pathophysiology content.[10] This is exactly why every component of what you do from day one is extremely important. Any concepts you brush over or short-term memorize may never be truly learned.

- Define your resources when preparing for this test. Without endorsing one resource over the other, there are key components that most successful US and non-US students use: question banks, video resources, study aids and reviews books such as First Aid for the USMLE. Despite all these, one study of students enrolled in US schools showed that academic performance and financial need may predict Step 1 score performance. Featuring eighty-four medical students at one institution in Florida, the students with the highest financial need performed lower than their counterparts without these needs. To that effect, those who utilized question banks and scored higher on the Comprehensive Basic Science Exams (CBSE) and USMLE world question banks performed better on the USMLE than the students who did

---

10 Adv Physiol Educ. 2014 Dec;38(4):315-20. doi: 10.1152/ advan.00047.2014

not. There was a correlation between the CBSE performance right before Step 1 and actual performance on the USMLE Step 1. Though not an endpoint, it also showed that spending longer studying did not correlate with improved performance on the test.[11] My deduction from that study is that you should test yourself using a test such as those created by the NBME prior to sitting for the real exam. In my opinion, you should not sit for the USMLE until you achieve a competitive score on the mock test.

- Set targets. There are three targets you will need: **score target**, **time-frame target**, and **schedule target**.

Score target. This is dependent on the specialty you choose to apply to. Using sample data from the 2019 match, the higher the score the better your chances at matching. One of the most frequently asked questions I receive is this: "What score do I need to get into residency?" My response is that it depends on the specialty you're interested in. I strongly encourage that you take a look at the NRMP's website.[12] Each year, they publish a graph showing the average scores that the matched and unmatched IMG category (US

11 Giordano C, Hutchinson D, Peppler R. A Predictive Model for USMLE Step 1 Scores. *Cureus*. 2016;8(9):e769. Published 2016 Sep 7. doi:10.7759/cureus.769

12 https://www.nrmp.org/wp-content/uploads/2018/06/Charting-Outcomes-in-the-Match-2018-Seniors.pdf

and non-US IMG) had during the cycle. This helped me deduce what the "acceptable average scores" were for each specialty, though this is not the intention for this curve. Unfortunately, these graphs cannot be reproduced without permission, but you can find them here: https://www.nrmp.org/wp-content/uploads/2018/06/Charting-Outcomes-in-the-Match-2018-Seniors.pdf.

The rule of thumb in the IMG community has always been to target a three-digit score above 240 as a safe zone. For the year 2018, across all specialties, the highest proportion of students (US and non-US IMGs) that matched had one thing in common: a higher score within this range. In my opinion, this makes this score target valid.

Time-frame target. The most common misconception in this process is that the longer you study, the better your performance on the USMLE. Personal experience and research disprove this. The number of days studying does not always correlate with your scores.[13] This is particularly true because, as mentioned in the previous chapter, Step 1 preparation begins during the basic science years.

Schedule target. You should have two schedules: one for your medical school curriculum and comprehensive exam, aka NBME prep, and a dedicated study period preparation. A dedicated

13 https://www.ncbi.nlm.nih.gov/pmc/articles/PMC5059149/

study period is crucial and should mimic the test. Most people who fail this test do so due to a lack of focus and tenacity for a very long exam.

CHAPTER 6

Pearls for the Clinical Years

Dr. Kim

I made the long drive (twelve hours STRAIGHT!) from Milwaukee to Atlanta to officially start my clinical rotations. I was excited! I was going to live with my brother, and I was excited to live in a major city with lots of celebrities and things to do. Maybe I would meet one of the Real Housewives?

My rotation in Atlanta was great: my peds rotation was split into three weeks in the Neonatal Intensive Care Unit (NICU) and three weeks in the clinic.

I learned a lot, met some other Caribbean medical students, although I, unfortunately, did not meet a Real Housewife. But I did meet another reality TV star!

I did most of my cores in Janesville, Wisconsin after doing pediatrics in Atlanta and staying with my brother. I had a pretty good experience. Other than my family medicine rotation (which was with residents and attendings), I was one-on-one with an attending. I was able to carry out a lot of procedures—especially on my surgery rotation—was able to help run clinics, and got to ask a lot of in-depth questions. Because I worked so closely with my attendings, I was able to ask for great letters of recommendation later down the road.

Rotations as a Caribbean student can be a mixed bag. Some places are focused on academics and are used to having students (international and US alike). Some places will not be used to you as a student. They may have lots of questions about your experience, your education, and your home country. The clinical experience that you receive may likely vary.

Here are a few tips on making the best out of your clinical years:

- **As always, failing to plan is planning to fail**. While you're awaiting your Step scores (and enjoying a break), do some research to find out the best places to get rotations. No matter what specialty you think you're interested in, your core rotations are crucial and will be foundational to your Step 2. Having a good clinical experience can augment study materials.

- **Try to do all, or most, of your cores in one location (hospital or city).** Ross called these tracks (all cores) or mini-tracks (some cores). Doing all of your cores in one location can save time and money since there are minimal gaps in the schedule. It can significantly decrease the time for finding short-term housing. The downside to doing all of your cores in one place is that you won't have the benefit of varied clinical experience from different parts of the country and hospital types. For example, if you do your cores in a big city with a big tertiary-care hospital, you may miss out on the types of patients that tend to come to smaller community hospitals. As you go through clinicals, you'll also learn that there are different practice patterns depending on what part of the country you're in. This can be due to culture, availability of resources, or how the hospitals are run. Experiencing variety in how people practice can help you shape your own practice in the future.

- **Read, read, read!** Find an interesting case from the day and read up on it. This will help solidify the medicine in your mind and help you study for Step 2.

- **Are you doing practice questions?** As a 3rd year medical student, you should know that the practice questions will never end. Even as I was preparing for my specialty boards, I was working and doing practice questions. You're likely preparing for an NBME Subject Examination (otherwise known as Shelf exams) at the end of a rotation. It's important to do practice questions regularly to know exactly what material the test will likely cover. I recommend UWorld for Step 2, but there may be some other question banks that you can go through to help you prep for boards.

- **Ask to make an oral presentation on a topic.** Taking a deep dive into a topic you may not know much about can be helpful in studying for Step 2. As well, oral presentations (as a PowerPoint) can be placed on your CV and will look great as you apply to residency.

- **Speaking of CV, you should be building it as you go through your clinicals.** Try to carve some time to volunteer and to find research opportunities. Make sure that you update your CV with every opportunity that you complete. This will make your life so much easier when you're compiling materials for your residency application.

- **Join the organization of your intended specialty and consider getting involved.**

Showing interest in your intended specialty by becoming a part of the college is something you can put on your CV. Students are often given FREE or deeply discounted membership rates and lots of opportunities to become involved in a national or international way.

Moreover, networking and mentorship are crucial for IMGs. Becoming a part of your intended specialty's organization affords you opportunities to mix, mingle, and network with your future colleagues. It also puts you into a position to seek and find a mentor that will help you match when the season comes around. Not a member of your future specialty's organization? Then put this book down— right now—open your computer and join today. Yes, it's *that* important.

- ***Practice, practice, practice* your assessment and plans.** Most third-year medicals know how to gather a great history and perform a physical exam exceptionally well. What sets students apart is when they start to think like their resident/attending. After you see your patient, pretend as though you are the sole physician taking care of the patient. What does this patient need today? What potential complications are you concerned about? Can the patient do their ADLs (activities of daily living)? Is there a new problem that has arisen? What complications may arise? By thinking about these things, you'll show that you're more than just a regular third-year medical student.

- **Write down any interesting or rare cases that you are a part of.** You can present these as posters at conferences or write up a case report to be published in a journal. Either way, this is a great way to build your CV.

- **Don't be afraid of not knowing something.** Rounding for hours on the floors and being pimped can be exhausting. If your attending or resident asks you something and you don't know the answer, it's okay to say that you don't know. You have a responsibility to your patients, but, thankfully, not all of the burden is on your shoulders. You are there to learn and do your best. But *go find the answer.* Whether it's something like how much oxygen your patient is on or describing the pathophysiology behind syncope in aortic stenosis, *go find the answer.*

- **Make friends with nurses and techs.** Many schools require you to have a certain number of procedures under your belt and you're required to keep a procedure log. Many procedures, doctors don't routinely perform; it's nurses or other medical professionals that may do them. IVs, nasogastric tubes, and Foley catheters should be a staple for all medical students. I got the most opportunities while I was on my surgery rotation.

- **Follow your patient to procedures.** On my

internal medicine rotations, I made a point to go down to interventional radiology to watch lumbar punctures, or to the cath lab to watch the cardiologist perform a cath. Learning about what actually happens when people have procedures done is not only beneficial to your learning but you can help explain things to your patients later down the road.

Dr. Nina

I swear I never had a migraine headache until my first clinical rotation as a third-year student. After surviving a long gap preparing for the USMLE and, more importantly, transitioning from Cameroon back to the States to begin clinical rotations in Chicago, I was so excited that I became anxious. In usual fashion, I had read all the blogs on clinicals, the what-to-dos, and the what-not-to-dos. I guess I had no idea that the wards were actually going to fill me with life and keep me invigorated.

My clinical years are the most beautiful of this entire phase. I strongly recommend that you embark on clinicals after you have successfully completed USMLE Step 1. This is the expectation for US medical students as well. Remember your goal is to mimic them so that your CV looks similar to theirs when it comes to residency application season. With the wave of new Caribbean schools popping up on almost every island, I have met a few students who completed all clinical rotations prior to sitting for Step 1! This is not the proper way to do this: remember that if you choose to go to a foreign medical school that mirrors the US medical education system, your school should actually do just that. Once you begin to deviate from the acceptable US standard, you can expect to begin to create a nontraditional path for yourself; medicine, as a whole, does not like nontraditional. Some argue that a pictorial idea of clinical work is essential in understanding some components of the structure of the questions you encounter during the USMLE boards. This is partially true, but the basic sciences, Step 1, then the clinical format has been tried and proven to be successful for many years now.

This book is about sharing my advice, so here you go.

- Begin seeking out audition rotations early enough (at the start of third year).

- Seek to do your core rotations at hospitals with affiliated teaching programs for the highest-quality education.

- If you are interested in a particular specialty, seek out opportunities that expose you to clinical chairs, department leaders, and even residency program directors of these specialties.

- If you are uncertain about what specialty to choose, do yourself a favor and seek to rotate through or shadow as many physicians as possible. You may never know what you like until you are exposed to it.

- Another great resource for getting exposure to other specialties is social media. There are several ways to see "a day in the life" of just about any specialty these days with the diverse mentorship platforms geared towards various groups.

- Attend conferences. And when you do, your

primary goals should be to present a poster and to network.

- Networking is key for the IMG. Especially for those who have gaps or are nontraditional, you may need a little more help than your counterparts. Meet programs and faculty, interact and showcase your interest.

- Do not accept being a spectator at a conference! Meet presenters, talk to programs in the vendor halls—they are there to meet you.

CHAPTER 7

Applying for Residency

Dr. Kim

I think ERAS crashes every year! September 15, 2014, while sitting in my room at a family friend's house, I woke up early to submit my application. I just had a night shift on my last rotation of medical school ever (emergency medicine!). I'd worked on my application for several weeks, arranged for my letters of recommendation and Standard Letters of Evaluation (SLOEs) to be submitted.

I was READY.

After I said a silent prayer to calm my nerves, I hit the submit button. I got an error. I tried to submit again.

No luck. OF COURSE, ERAS is down! Apparently, ERAS wasn't ready for me, or all the other students frantically trying to submit their applications. Talk about frustrated! I think I almost had a meltdown worried that this was going to negatively affect my application.

Spoiler alert: I was able to submit the next day—no harm, no foul ☺.

From before I got my acceptance letter into Ross until submitting my ERAS application, emergency medicine was ingrained into my mind. After spending time in the Ecuadorian equivalent of the emergency department, I knew that EM was the specialty I was looking for. I also had a background in public health, and emergency medicine to me was the essence of public health. I would literally take care of anyone and everyone who walked through the doors, no matter what. Throughout my time in medical school, I truly enjoyed something from every core rotation and I loved doing procedures, no matter how small. My surgery rotation was full of starting nasogastric tubes, Foley catheters, IVs, checking surgical incisions, being the first or second assist on cases, taking sutures and staples out in surgery clinic. During obstetrics and gynecology, I loved talking to future moms in the clinic, measuring their fundal height, checking for fetal heart tones, and being the first person to touch a new human entering this world. During my psychiatry rotation, I was fascinated by how schizophrenia and bipolar disorder revealed itself in my patients, and how they progressively got better as we put them on medication. Emergency medicine would be the blend of every specialty and I was excited.

With that being said, of course everyone isn't as clear about their specialty choice. If you're stuck, here are some things to consider:

- Take a full inventory of yourself. What do you like inside of medicine? What hobbies or passions do you have outside of medicine? What do you generally like and not like?

- Ask yourself what you see yourself doing over the next twenty-plus years into your career.

- What would your perfect day at work be?

- Do you like to work independently or as a team?

- Surgery vs medicine? Or a blend of both?

- Is there any specialty you completely dislike or love?

- If you couldn't do your number-one specialty, is there another specialty (or two) that you'd be happy in?

- What is it about your chosen specialty that makes you excited?

- Is there a certain population you want to serve?

Women? Children? The elderly?

Asking yourself the tough questions will help guide you into the right specialty to apply to. As well, *every IMG should have a backup specialty*, especially if they are applying to a competitive one.

Once you've solidified your specialty, and backup specialty, applying needs to be extremely strategic. While you are sprucing up your CV, writing your personal statement, and gathering letters of recommendation, you'll need to strategize which programs you'll apply to.

If you are born in the US, you have a better chance of obtaining a stateside residency because you will not need a visa. However, if you were born outside the US, this may be a significant hurdle. Regardless of where your citizenship lies, you'll need to narrow down programs that will be the most friendly to you as an IMG.

The best ways to find IMG friendly programs are:

- **Caribbean medical schools' websites.** Schools publish a match list of where their graduates match for residency. Look at all of the "Big Four" (Ross University, American University of the Caribbean, Saba, and St. George's) schools match lists and apply to every program that you can where someone has matched.

- **Online message boards and forums** are a

great way to hear about new programs that are opening up for the match. New programs can be more open to IMGs.

- **Tools like Match a Resident.** By taking your Step scores and other data, they can make a personalized list of where you'll have the highest likelihood of matching. This service does have a fee. I'm a proponent of making your list without paying any service to help you; however, if you are not a US citizen, Match a Resident can be helpful in sorting through programs that will take a visa.

Speaking of money, budgeting is key. This is another time in your medical career where there will be a significant financial investment (as if the USMLEs weren't enough!). Before ERAS accepts your application, you can see exactly how much you may be charged to apply to a certain number of programs. Try your best to balance your budget with how many programs you apply to. Keep in mind that you will actually have to travel to some of these places when interviews begin to roll in.

Once you actually submit your ERAS application, there is a lot of waiting around, refreshing your email multiple times a day expecting an interview invite to come in.

Here are some tips to actually obtain interviews:

- **ASK!** If it's been several weeks and you still

haven't heard from a program, it's okay to reach out to programs and express interest. This can be done with a polite email to the program director or program coordinator (with your ERAS # in the signature) or a polite phone call. It's also appropriate to express your interest in the program specifically, whether it's the location, fellowship opportunities, a special focus for residents, or whatever piques your fancy about it. Showing your interest in what the program has to offer shows that you are interested in going there specifically.

- **NETWORK!** I went to multiple emergency medicine conferences during my third and fourth year of medical school. During application season, I attended the American College of Emergency Physicians (ACEP) Scientific Assembly and actually met my program director in person (rare … more on that in the next chapter) and received an invite a day later! Although this is NOT how most people get interviews, networking at major specialty conferences can set you apart from the sea of applicants to your program. Keep in touch with those that you meet.

- **Online forums and message boards.** By using sites such as Student Doctor Network, I knew when others started receiving interview invitations and could start strategizing when I would reach out to my top programs. I could also see others' impressions of the programs as well.

DR. NINA

There was no defined thought or moment that led to how I chose a specialty to apply to. For me, the "law of environment" led me to primary care. At the beginning of this chapter, Dr. Kim laid out pertinent questions to consider when choosing a specialty. I believe there is not much else to add to that.

I am not proud of how I applied for residency, but, in many ways, it has been one of the key reasons I started coaching IMGs. Simply put, I was entirely clueless about what I was doing. I spent the majority of my clinical rotations without variety. What I mean by this is I focused on rotating at a hospital that had multiple rotations to offer but only one ACGME (Accreditation Council for Graduate Medical Education) approved program and this was in family medicine.

In the context of the previous chapter, I became very familiar with how the FM residency process worked as a result of the time spent at this hospital. I was fully ingrained into it. My preceptors and those I looked up to were all FM board certified. It was an easy choice based on my indirect influences. Based on my environment, I was exposed to one specialty and my application portfolio (curriculum vitae, clinical experiences, presentation, research) were all geared towards primary care. This is where the law of the environment comes into play. If you want to develop into a particular specialty, it is in your best interests to rotate, shadow, and seek out clinical experiences in that specialty. What you are doing is building a suitable portfolio that shows you are interested in that discipline above all the others.

Remember, you will only produce based on the environment you cultivate in. This is why, if you are remotely interested in a specialty, I *strongly* urge you to seek a mentor in that same specialty and spend all your free time with them to learn from their experiences.

Next step, when it comes to applying into residency, I recommend you use a filtering resource. There are several programs available on the internet that will allow you to input specific elements, such as year of graduation, specialty of interest, Step 1 score, and visa requirement (just to name a few). This will then auto-populate a list of possible eligible programs for you to follow.

If you do not want to pay for such a resource, then remember the AMA provides a free database known as the FREIDA Residency Program. I was reading today on the AMA's website and found some pretty amazing statistics on the number of positions open during a recent match cycle. Below, you can see the total number of available first-year positions across the country, according to the FREIDA Residency Program Database in 2019, although this does not include specialties like ophthalmology, urology, dermatology, orthopedics, radiation–oncology, plastic surgery, neurosurgery, etc. When reviewing this information below, note that a categorical position provides full residency training required for board certification in that specialty, whereas a preliminary position offers one-to-two years of training prior to entering an advanced specialty program.

- Internal medicine: 11,515 first-year residency positions (including preliminary positions)

- Family medicine: 4,890 first-year residency positions

- Pediatrics: 3,226 first-year positions

- Surgery—general: 2,868 first-year residency positions (including preliminary positions)

- Emergency medicine: 2,739 first-year residency positions

- Psychiatry: 1,906 first-year residency positions

- Anesthesiology: 1,679 first-year residency positions

- Transitional year: 1,653 first-year residency positions

- Obstetrics and gynecology: 1,512 first-year residency positions

- Radiology—diagnostic: 1,187 first-year residency positions

Though not all-inclusive, I share these numbers to show you that all you need is one spot, one chance, one shot!

Newsflash: guess what …?

You can only fill one spot at a time!

Statistics show that most IMGs choose to practice within one of the above specialties but there are some that practice even within specialties traditionally considered to be more competitive. So do not shortchange yourself! You have to define your goals for yourself independent of statistics. You own the stats because you can create a new denominator! If you work hard and dedicate yourself wholeheartedly to the pursuit of your goal, I bet there has to be one of these thousands of positions that is yours for a period of at least three to five years. Better believe it.

Experience being the best teacher, consider talking with doctors who have been where you want to be. They are more likely to reveal the best advice that pertains to their individual specialty. As an example, on my blog, drninalum.com, I interviewed IMGs that matched into even the more competitive specialties, and in that process I learned that certain specialties cherish particular research experience more than others. That makes a difference between what is an absolute requirement in ophthalmology versus psychiatry. When it comes to fellowship, my theory is that once you get into residency, everything else is possible because you are essentially in the door. If you are interested in learning from the successes of others, I suggest you read and listen to the stories on my blog series titled "The IMG Roadmap Series." You can find this on drninalum.com. Another great resource is my podcast of the same title, which is available on Apple podcasts, Google podcasts and wherever else you listen to your favorite podcasts. You will not regret soaking up in all this advice from other IMGs.

CHAPTER 8

Interview Season

Dr. Kim

I *KNEW* that Memphis was going to be the place for me. Crossing over the bridge from Arkansas into Tennessee, I could feel that THIS was going to be right. As I entered the city, I could see my potential training hospitals, and I excitedly showed each of them to my mom, who was driving with me.

Prior to submitting my ERAS application, I'd emailed my (future) program director after finding out on a message board that the program would be opening. After returning to the States, I decided that I wanted to try my best to do my residency in the south, preferably in Tennessee. I'd completed my undergrad in Tennessee and it had become a home away from home. So, after hearing about a new program in Memphis, I leaped at the opportunity to find out more information. My Google searching came up with no website or information regarding the program. I called the hospital's emergency department to find out if the rumors were true. I was then directed to my (future) program director and received his email address. We emailed back and forth, and I found out that he would be at the ACEP annual conference. I made a point to meet him in person.

Fast forward some weeks after my ERAS application was submitted, I was at ACEP participating in the medical student track. There was a luncheon where program directors went around to different tables and shared information about their program. The very first program to come to my table was ... the program director from Memphis. Immediately after the luncheon, I tracked him down and spoke to him again, reminding him of who I was and that I'd emailed him a few months prior. I expressed my sincere interest in the program, including its newness, its critical-care opportunities, and the proximity to family and friends from my college years. A day later, I received an interview invite to come to Memphis.

The pre-interview experience was great. Since the program was brand new and matching their first class, future faculty members sat with us as interviewees.

Dinner was delicious, and I had a great time getting to know the future faculty. We laughed and joked around the entire evening. It felt very natural and comfortable. I left the dinner and told my mom, "This is it … I just know it!"

Interview day started early, and I had a tour of the emergency department and great interviews with two of the same faculty members that were at dinner the night before. We picked up the conversation from the previous night, and they asked me about my experience at Fisk University, which is world-renowned for the Fisk Jubilee Singers.

I left the experience feeling energized and excited.

Now, of course that story was all roses and tulips. And spoiler alert, I ranked Memphis number one and matched there. However, I had other experiences that were not as warm and fuzzy. Several times on the trail, I was the only Caribbean graduate in the room with other interviewees. Sometimes, it felt intimidating. I questioned, "Am I really supposed to be here?"

Regardless, interview season is actually fun. Traveling around, meeting new people, possibly bumping into people you already know, is exciting. It's one thing to read everything possible about a program on a website, but to physically be there is another.

I was also surprised at how relaxed the interviews generally were. Most interviewers will not grill you about why you got a certain grade in a subject back on the island. By the time you are sitting in the interview chair, they already like you. They want to see if you're a good fit for that specific program. All program directors want someone *personable* and *teachable*.

Here are some tips based on my experiences:

- **Networking is invaluable.** Of course, I was able to network my way into an interview at my number-one program, but don't forget to network with other interviewees. I ran into someone I interviewed with while I was taking my oral board exam. The world is small; you never know where you'll end up or who you'll meet along the way.

- **If you're early, you're on time. If you're on time, you're late.** So many interview days start way early in the morning (7 a.m.). If you're anything like me (read: NOT a morning person), do everything in your power to make sure you are up, bright and ready to go the morning of. Pick a hotel as close to the interview location as possible, set multiple alarms, lay out your clothes and accessories the night before so there's no rush.

- **Utilize all of the travel perks and discount websites you can.** Traveling will get expensive, quickly. Strongly consider only bringing a carryon if flying. As well, consider other options for travel like bus or train, which may be cheaper than flying. I took the train from Milwaukee to St. Louis for an interview. Not only was it cheaper than flying, I enjoyed the experience of traveling in a different way than I had before. Plus, when you're interviewing in the Midwest during the winter, there's a lower likelihood that a train would be behind schedule or canceled.

- **Be professional but show your personality.** Wear your favorite color in your shirt or socks. Discuss your love for sports, hiking, basket weaving, opera singing (true story), what have you. You're unique, and expressing what you like sets you apart from the rest. Plus, you may have an interviewer that's interested in what you like as well.

- **Consider staying a few extra hours, rather than leaving town immediately after the interview (if you can afford it).** Staying just a little longer can allow you to explore the city, to trying out some great restaurants. Or just take a mini-vacation! On an interview I had in Detroit, Michigan, I stayed an hour or so after the interview day to take a look at the residents at work. That extra time I spent allowed me to get a better feel for the program, and I realized that that program would likely not be a good fit for me. My short time investment helped me to prioritize my rank-order list down the road.

Dr. Nina

My first interview remains a bit of a freezing blur. It was in Michigan somewhere ... It was cold! I remember taking a train from Chicago to Michigan the night before. There was no fancy dinner, no pre-interview. The entire day itself felt as scary as being pushed into Lake Michigan in twenty-degree weather in the middle of December. I do not remember much of the interview day itself, even though I only interviewed at two places.

One thing I do remember about this season was that my visa requirement posed a great hindrance. For students with visa requirements, I strongly recommend that you consider applying to many more programs than the average US person. This is because there are only a limited number of programs that will sponsor a visa. This automatically limits your chances of matching by default, so, for whatever chances remain, you want to cast a really wide net.

You can rely on some states to be generally more IMG friendly than others. Based on data from the NRMP, the more friendly ones include (but are not limited to) New York, Michigan, Pennsylvania, Florida, Texas, New Jersey, Illinois, and Ohio. Be cautious, though, not to limit yourself to only these states because, as you will find out in real life, there are IMGs in Wyoming and Maine too! Well, without going too far away, I matched in Kentucky, while Dr. Kim did so in Tennessee! By inference too, there are many programs located in the NY/NJ area when compared with the KY/TN area.

Moral: You can make an IMG friendly program if you are a good fit.

Back to the interview trail. I applied in October, something I would not recommend any IMG to do. I always recommend that due to the competitive nature of the application process these days, it is important to be ready from the beginning. Programs have a lot of information to filter through and there are other candidates (i.e., your competition) who are going to apply as soon as ERAS opens, with complete application packets and great scores. For example, my friend Dr. F, who is currently on faculty at a family medicine program, informed me that at her program's incomplete IMG applications are kept in a holding bin that may never get revisited if the interview slots are filled up with interested candidates who have completed applications. You have to be participating in the race to win it, right?

Well, so it was now the end of October, and I was not receiving any interview invitations. This was in 2011 when the rules were less stringent. So I took a day off to sit down at home and comb through my list. I researched the telephone numbers of all the programs I applied to. I started from the top and called them up, one right after the other. I mostly fell on the program coordinator's voicemail but I did not stop. I kept calling. These calls resulted in one more interview. This time in Kentucky. At this point, you know how that story ends. My advice to you is to do whatever is legally, professionally, and ethically appropriate to get you acknowledged by the program you desire to match into.

Dr. Kim already laid out some ideas as to how to gain interviews. I think the easiest interviews to get are those at programs where you previously rotated as a medical student. That makes a huge difference because these programs know you and have spent a lot of time with you to determine early on whether you will be a good fit for them. But here are a few pointers for interview day itself.

- Keep your appearance professional, conservative, and neutral. Wear comfortable, closed-toe shoes.

- Prepare answers for the most frequently asked questions you expect to receive during the interview. You can find these on the internet for just about every specialty that exists.

- Practice, practice, practice! This is most effective when you practice with someone who has been on the other side of where you are now—meaning you should consider practicing with either a resident or an attending you admire that is doing exactly what you want to be doing in the future.

- Always carry a copy of your resume and your personal statement with you on the official interview date as most interviewers ask questions based on what you previously revealed about yourself.

- Be prompt, make eye contact, show and express an interest in what you are interviewing for! Remember to be kind to everyone you meet— they all have a role to play, even the coordinators and residents.

- After the interview, I strongly recommend that you leave a line of communication open. What this means is do consider sending a thank-you note or email to the faculty members/residents you met. Yes, even to the program coordinator (we now know they are the backbone of most of the administrative duties of most teaching programs). This will allow interested parties to respond.

- Another strategic time to communicate with programs is right before the rank list is submitted. Usually, this can serve as a reminder that you are still interested in training at your facility of interest.

Now onto the topic of visas, for non-US IMGs. You want to focus on programs that sponsor visas. There are two major types of visa classes applicable here. One is the Student Exchange Visitor Visa, aka J-1 Visa, and the other is the H1B, aka work visa. Both have pathways that lead to the holder potentially becoming eligible for a permanent residency card. In my opinion, this process seems to favor physicians. As a previous holder of the J-1 Visa category, I am well familiar with it. Its greatest limitation is the condition upon which it is founded. It requires the holder to return to their home country for two years or to serve in a US medically underserved area for three years upon completion of residency. Please verify with the USCIS (United States Citizenship and Immigration Service) as laws do change. In my experience, most US academic institutions, especially state universities, always seem to have a sponsorship program for J-1 Visa candidates. There is also some evidence that most fellowship programs prefer the J-1 Visa over the H1B Visa. The H1V visa does not carry the mandatory service requirement I just mentioned. During my time, successful completion of the USMLE (United States Medical Licensure Examination) step 3 was required to qualify for this visa type. Most non-US IMGs appreciate the liberty to choose the location of their employer. This alone has made the H1B visa more desirable.

CHAPTER 9

The Match

DR. KIM

By January, my interviews had slowed down significantly, and I was ready to rank my programs. As I went along the interview trail, I knew which programs I liked and those that would be lower on my list, so I basically made my rank-order list as the season went by.

To solidify my interest in Memphis, I decided to go back for a second look, contacting an attending that I had a good rapport with on my interview day. My second look went well. I saw a patient having STEMI , watched an off-service resident do a central line, and watched a lumbar puncture. In the middle of the shadow shift, I told my attending directly that I wanted to be there, and I was ranking them #1.

I had my top programs UT-Memphis, University of Kansas, and Sinai Grace. I sent them all emails informing them I intended on ranking them highly, or in the case of Memphis, that I was ranking them #1.

I submitted and finalized my list and tried to forget about it.

But I couldn't. I had interviewed at eight emergency medicine programs and three internal medicine programs, one of which had already offered me a position outside of the match. I declined it. I hoped I wouldn't have to dip into my backup specialty.

Then I questioned my rank list. I really liked Kansas. I wish I had gone back for a second look there, but my budget wouldn't allow it. I had family in the Memphis area, and I made the decision from finances and a gut feeling.

Monday of Match Week finally rolled around after what seemed like an excruciating six weeks. I couldn't even enjoy my birthday the month before because I was so anxious about matching. When the email rolled in, I held my breath. I HAD MATCHED! I decided that I would party all week long! Well, it was St. Patrick's Day week. On Friday, I matched into my number-one program, UT-Memphis! Around 1 p.m., my program director called to welcome and congratulate me and let me know who else would be in my class. I was on cloud nine.

I realize now that I had several advantages in matching the very first try:

- Being a US citizen

- Being from a "big four" Caribbean medical school

- No failed attempts at USMLE and improvement from Step 1 to Step 2

Even if you don't fit into any of those categories, you can also have a successful match story.

- Make sure, before you interview, you have taken USMLE Step 1, 2CS, and CK.

- Make sure everything is on track for you to be ECFMG certified. This is important to have before you begin residency on July 1.

- Make your rank list based on things that are truly important to you. The match leans on your preferences.

- Rank every program that extended you an interview. Most IMGs would rather match to their least preferred program, rather than not match at all. If there is a reason that you leave a program off your list, it should only be because, in the worst-case scenario, you'd prefer not to match at all.

- Make sure to certify your rank list before the last day! ***If it's not certified, you will not be entered into the match process***. After certification, you can still make changes, before the deadline.

- If you have doubts, and can afford it, ask for a second look at a program that piqued your interest. Spending some time with the residents and faculty outside of the formal interview setting can help solidify or bring to light things that you wouldn't have previously known about.

Dr. Nina

The match process for me was straightforward. I only had two programs to rank. I sent out thank-you emails to both programs, and I sort of knew which one of them was going to rank me. Seeing as all I heard back from the Michigan program were "crickets," I knew there was a lower likelihood that I would make the rank list, so I ranked them second. But something was different about Kentucky. They emailed me out of the blue one day to ask about my preference with an anticipated change in the intern year schedule. For some odd reason, I took that to be a sign that I was at least getting considered for a higher spot on the rank list. And I was!

For students who get invited to interview at several programs, creating the rank list can be a challenge. The US NRMP match process follows an algorithm where each program creates a list of preferred candidates by order of preference. Each student or graduate also creates a list of programs by order of preference. If both the program and the candidate align closely with one another, there is a higher probability of matching. The caveat, though, is these programs are not allowed to disclose your position on the rank list prior to the results. This leaves the candidate uncertain, especially if there has been little-to-no communication since the interview date. As a student, you will likely wonder which program will rank you high, then you try to rank them equally high; but, at the same time, you may like another program even though you are not certain how they perceived your interview experience with them. This can be confusing, but the usual adage goes: rank the programs you know you want to train at. To that, I would add that if you completely messed up the interview and it became very apparent that you were less desirable or undesirable to the program, then you should only rank them if that is really where you want to go.

Match day was the most anxiety-provoking day of my life! My American visa, which allowed me to participate in clinical rotations, was about to expire. Considering I was an off-cycle student due to the gap I had before taking USMLE Step 1, I completed my fourth-year clinical rotations at the end of January of 2012 (the same year I was enrolled in the match and the same year I would eventually start residency training). It was set to expire on March 30, 2020. So there I was, in the middle of the month, about to face a life-changing moment. I was scheduled to depart from the United States on March 30: my ticket was ready, my family was ready on the other side of the world to receive me in Douala, Cameroon.

Uncertainty pervaded through me. "What if I don't match?" was a recurring question every morning. I imagined myself going home at the end of the month … with either a victorious dance or a walk of shame and regret.

"Who leaves home to study abroad to return without

what they went there for?" The questions in my head were numerous.

Noon on match day may as well be the day and time that the gates of hell open up! That is when the NRMP traditionally updates the website to share the results for those of us who do not have match day rallies at our respective schools.

I found myself on a swing, in full regression, like a child waiting for an opportunity to either celebrate or cry my eyes out. The email came … And here I am today, writing this book, reminiscing that moment in time like it wasn't mine. The worry … Was it so necessary? I don't know for sure, but I can say I do not think so. It was such a stressful time, though: the visa hurdles, severely limited finances, amounting student loan debt, my odds of future success, the stress of difficult examinations. All these stressors mounted up against me for four-plus years, but in the end, I made it to the other side as an attending physician. You can do the same and even better!

But I also believe that fear of failure helped me work hard during medical school. It helped me hustle and it made me come out of my comfort zone to network, to smile, to talk to people and interact in ways that were outside of my usual. In the end, I do know hard work pays off, that perseverance conquers difficulties. If you hold on to faith and do not give up on your dreams, you will be amazed where you will end up.

CHAPTER 10

Still MD : Intern Year and Beyond

Dr. Kim

July 1, 2015, I walked into Methodist University Hospital in Memphis, TN as a brand new emergency medicine resident. I had on my brand new gray scrubs and a black fleece jacket that I got while I was rotating on trauma surgery at the famous Cook County Hospital. My nervousness was compounded because, two days prior, I had totaled my car after leaving a coffee date with a friend. I was really sad about my car and worried about how I was going to get around a new city without one.

On top of that, I was nervous and excited about actually starting residency, but luckily, I didn't have a shift on the first day. July 4 was when the action started for me, and my first shift was nothing short of crazy! We had a trauma arrest, a patient complaining of shortness of breath—which was a large pleural effusion that needed a chest tube—and much more craziness. It was a miracle that I made it through the night! A few days later, I was working another shift when they paged overhead, "I need a doctor to Room 22!" I was a doctor, right? I also happened to be sitting near Room 22. When I walked in, I found someone having a seizure and bleeding from their femoral artery. I froze for a second. *What in the WORLD?!* I had absolutely no idea how to help ... I rushed out of the room to get an attending. After Dr. Huggins came in, he directed someone to hold pressure on the bleeding, started an IV to give some anti-seizure medicine, and prepared to intubate the patient.

Was this what I had signed up for?

My first few months as an intern were challenging in so many different ways. Clinically, the patients were extremely medically complex. Was emergency medicine like this everywhere? Had I made a mistake coming to Memphis? I'm sure every intern has these thoughts at some point. I doubted myself way earlier. Looking back, my uncertainties about myself as an intern were likely a combination of things, like being a Caribbean grad, the only resident of color, and one of two female residents. As well, we were the first class of residents to go through the program. I had no upper-level residents to look to for guidance. As time progressed, though, I realized that I was just as prepared with medical knowledge as my co-residents, even though I was educated outside of the US.

Academically, I never had an issue in medical school or residency after my very first semester at Ross. Ross gave me the tools to learn how to study in order to prepare for clinical knowledge and standardized testing. I performed as well as my classmates in all of my in-service exams. Those same skills have carried me through to becoming board certified in emergency medicine. Throughout my residency, I presented research at regional conferences, served on hospital committees to improve emergency department processes, and overall, tried to significantly contribute to the hospital and the patients that we served.

DR. NINA

Intern year was actually quite exciting. Nothing could stop me! My whole life up to that moment had been for this. It was my turn to shine, to make up for all my mishaps. I was not going to let fear ruin it. Quickly after orientation, I realized that all interns were made equal. Ignorance knew no discrimination. Actually, where we went to school was never a topic of conversation. Matter of fact, I was surprised to find out about the other IMGs in my program later in the year. It did not matter one bit: we were all just trying to survive, trying to understand duty hours, and really just trying not to kill anyone. Oh, and did I forget, this was a true shot at our dreams? My life goals were manifesting—nothing could get in their way.

I am now a firm believer that the limitations we place on ourselves are entirely ours. The mind is a dynamic space: you can create success or failure within. It can create scenarios and contexts that do not really exist, ones that can trap you into a vortex of self-fabricated inferiority. Once I became an upper level supervising junior residents, I realized that all interns are truly made equal. To a certain extent, we are all green when we first start out, irrespective of how great a medical school we attended.

Residency training is the greatest learning opportunity of your career and your best shot to become the best physician you can possibly be. Take it at face value, give it your best effort. I realized that I could really learn what I wanted to know in medicine during this period. I chose to redefine myself, redefine my chances of success. Because guess what? We were all getting trained here in America and to the same standards. Due to the difficulties I faced as an international medical student, I was more resilient and found long workdays pleasurable. I was more thankful for the opportunities that led me to actually enjoy my work. There was no one day where I felt burnout as a resident. Despite the sleepless nights, schedule conflicts, lack of family time, etc., I still found daily things to be thankful for. For once as a true MD, walking in my dreams, I no longer felt subservient or ashamed of my past.

I began to develop in my style of practice and slowly realized that my hardships helped me build tenacity. My story began to change. I believed in myself more each day. So during the long days and the tough nights, all I could think of was how much I wanted this, how hard I worked, and, more importantly, how blessed I was to receive this gift of education and a gift to serve and heal others. Those days in Cameroon came full circle.

You may be reading this while waiting to begin your intern year, or maybe you are still waiting to match. I want you to know that you will only reap what you sow in each phase of your life. You should walk into residency expectant and adopt a growth mindset. Tell yourself things like "I am here to learn," "This is going to be the best educational season of my life thus far," "I have what it takes to make it," and "I am deserving of this opportunity." Change the internal rhetoric, beat that imposter syndrome. Feeling like a fraud will not advance your career; it will only hold you back!

CONCLUSION

Beyond the Blue Seas

DR. KIM

Now that I'm an attending, my days on the island seem like a distant past. Going to medical school in another country was a big challenge, which, looking back, made me a stronger and resilient person. I never thought I would be someone that would leave the comfort of my own country to pursue a lifelong dream ... and be successful at it. The unique opportunity of being educated outside of the US should be received with pride. Reflecting on my winding path to medicine, I wish I had taken the leap of faith to go to a Caribbean medical school sooner and not listened to others' negative perceptions.

When I was making the decision whether to apply to Caribbean schools or not, I wondered if my patients would perceive me differently or if people would be able to spot a difference between my education and another physician's education.

Guess what? No one can tell the difference. At the end of the day, you are still an MD.

Dr. Nina

I have met numerous phenomenal physicians and surgeons in real day practice from all the corners of the earth. This is the reason why I share their stories on my podcast titled "The IMG Roadmap Podcast". You can find it on my website www.drninalum.com, Apple Podcasts, Google Podcasts and wherever else you listen to your favorite stories. But on the IMG Roadmap Podcast, I empower, equip and encourage IMGs. I interview physicians who are thriving in medicine and surgery who just happened to have graduated from foreign medical schools. I do this because I want IMGs to continue to lead, heal and shine like they ought to. There is no reason for us (IMGs) to feel or function like second tier physicians when we are equally productive members of the US healthcare system. It has been my observation that what matters most is our productivity and the value we add to the healthcare system in America and across the world. Even among my coworkers, at the present time, there is no distinction between those who graduated from a school located outside of the US versus inside. There is no MD (Doctor of Medicine) versus DO (Doctor of Osteopathic medicine). We are all doctors, surgeons, physicians and medical professionals united on one front. Serving mankind. Saving lives. We all passed the respective board exams demonstrating expertise in our diverse specialties. There is a joke I do not like that keeps getting shared but if I had to flip it, it would read something like this:

Question: "What do you call a phenomenal doctor who graduated from a school outside of the mainland USA?"

Response: "Doctor."

This brings me to the affirmation that lies in the title of our book. In essence, affirming the physician whose path was slightly different and maybe required an expedition across the blue seas. I want you to know that you are not alone and that there are countless others who have gone before you to make the way clearer for you to follow. I hope you choose to believe in yourself and in your journey as much as I do. And for heaven's sake, just do the right thing! Stay focused, stay in school, complete medical school in four years, take the boards once (each time), seek out opportunities for audition rotations, perform research where applicable, apply smart, and watch things unfold in your favor!

BONUS

Advice from Other IMGs

"You have to believe in yourself and be able to advocate for yourself throughout this journey and in the end trust that you will be where you are supposed to be." — **Sharon Udemba, St. George's University, MS II**

"There is so much I want to say. However, I'll try to keep it short. What I have learned in my journey is the importance of staying focused, disciplined, and always asking questions. In addition to this, network, network, network ... Did I say 'network'? This could help you get through a door. Seek guidance from people that have been through your journey. Nobody will understand what you are going through better than the ones that have gone through it. Start early; time will fly by, and towards the end, you will have other things to worry about—do not procrastinate. Do your research, and whenever you fall off the wagon, don't beat yourself up. Times will come where you will want to give up. But don't. Get back on track and get back stronger. Make sure you have a tribe, circle that will encourage, push you, hold you accountable, a tribe that will celebrate your wins and comfort you during your losses, a tribe that will love and support you through it all. Please don't give up. keep pushing, you can do it! The Journey to MD—it's hard but worth it!" — **Valentina Oside, Washington University of Health Science, MS IV**

"Even though some people might look at you differently because you're an IMG, don't let that get to you. Be proud that you made the sacrifice to study abroad and accepted the challenge to study medicine in a foreign country. At the end of the day, location of studies is not what your patient will ask you or expect from you. They're going to expect good care. Also, the IMG community is large – always make those connections because you are not alone!" — **Melis Coklar, MS III, St. George's University, Grenada**

"As an international medical student, just realize that this is the journey that has been chosen for you. Do not compare your journey to others because it will not be the same. I am a mother of four, and I never thought I would be here, but I AM and I AM PROUD of MYSELF!" — **Nina Snowden, MS III**

"After you get your letter of admission, before you get on the plane to the island, buy a journal. On the first page write out your 'why'. Write out your 5-year plan and everything else you'd like to accomplish with this degree. This book will come in handy when things get difficult and you feel like giving up. Also, remember you have everything within you to be everything you want to be. Don't ever give up! The world needs you." — **Paula Nwajei, MD**, **All Saints School of Medicine (currently awaiting residency)**

Even though some people might look at you differently because you're an IMG, don't let that get to you. Be proud that you made the sacrifice to study abroad and accepted the challenge to study medicine in a foreign country. At the end of the day, location of studies is not what your patient will ask you or expect from you. They're going to expect good care. Also, the IMG community is large – always make those connections because you are not alone! — **Melis Coklar, MS III, St. George's University, Grenada**

ABOUT THE AUTHORS

Dr. Nina Lum

Dr. Nina Lum is a Hospitalist and the Chief Quality Officer at CHI St. Joseph Hospital in London, Kentucky. She is board certified in family medicine and has focused on hospital medicine practice since graduating from The University of Kentucky Rural Track/St. Claire Family Medicine in 2015, where she was the chief resident. At CHI St. Joseph London, she currently oversees quality and safety initiatives within the facility.

Dr. Lum was born in Douala, Cameroon. In 2012, she graduated from The University of Sint Eustatius School of Medicine (NKA American University of Integrative Sciences AUIS) in the Netherlands Antilles and moved to Kentucky in 2012 to pursue medical residency training.

She is a co-author of the best-selling medical

anthology "The Chronicles of Women in White Coats" and recently the visionary, co-creator and co-author of the Amazon bestseller "Beyond Challenges: Survival Stories of African Immigrant Physicians."

As the chief blogger on www.theencouragingdoc.com and www.drninalum.com she writes and coaches international medical students & graduates on success blueprints for their unique pathway. She is the creator of the online course-coaching platform for IMGs known as imgroadmap.com. She is a featured health & wellness speaker and previously was a newspaper columnist for Sentinel Echo. She has also been featured on WLEX and Fox 56.

Dr. Lum is also an avid medical missionary and has worked with teams in Haiti & Cameroon. She loves coaching others, media, photography, entrepreneurship, travel, blogging, and reading on self-improvement.

Website: www.drninalum.com
Instagram: @drninalum
Facebook: Nina Lum, MD

Dr. Kimberly Brown

Kimberly M. Brown, MD, MPH is a board-certified emergency physician and public health professional with a passion for health education and disease prevention. She is also the best-selling author of *It's an Emergency!: Understanding the What, How and Why of Your ER Visit*, is a speaker and media personality featured on Untold Stories of the ER, Local Memphis 24, Fox 13 Memphis, Health.com, Doximity, the Women in White Coats blog and podcast, and Medical Economics.

Born and raised in Milwaukee, Wisconsin, she left home to attend Fisk University, where she graduated magna cum laude with a Bachelor of Arts in Biology. She completed a Master of Public Health degree with a concentration in Public Health Management and Policy from the University of Florida. In 2014, she earned her Doctor of Medicine degree from Ross University School of Medicine. She completed her emergency medicine residency at the University of Tennessee Health Science Center in Memphis, Tennessee.

Dr. Brown currently lives, works, and plays in Memphis. She does her best writing in her bed, snuggled up under the covers and listening to podcasts. In her free time, she enjoys traveling, watching the Real Housewives, kickboxing, and spending time with her friends.

www.drkimberlyb.com
Facebook.com/drkimberlyb
Instagram: @drkimberlyb

CPSIA information can be obtained
at www.ICGtesting.com
Printed in the USA
BVHW030932120220
572157BV00001B/69